Understanding Medicare Part D

By: Chuck Robinson

Table of Contents

CHAPTER ONE

INTRODUCTION

> Customer: *"Why do they not have adult education classes for this?!?"*
>
> Me: *"I don't know sir, they should!" (**Thinking...Why don't I?)*

The first day of training at my new job I thought I was so behind. I am lucky if I can remember the difference between Medicare and Medicaid. Now I have a job with a Medicare prescription drug plan? How did I get myself into this?!

Well it turns out I was not at all alone. Most of my coworkers started on the exact same page. I quickly learned most people around me in my life were the same; my mom who was turning 64 was ecstatic I was going to be learning about this to help her sign up next year, and eventually I learned a majority of the people I helped on the phone each day were just as confused as I started out at. For an educated individual as myself, it was still hard for myself to comprehend. While some of my colleagues looked at our job as a "job", I couldn't turn a blind eye to what I was seeing. I don't believe these seniors are losing it but they must not be getting the right information. I kept saying this to myself this each night after work.

After a few years of talking on the phone with members I thought that there should be a much easier way to get this information into a format that is easier to understand. I hated hearing a customer that was frustrated with having to choose to medicine OR pay for their rent and food. Can you imagine getting a call from a sweet 70 year old woman from Florida, ordering medications and upon realizing the price, hearing her start to panic? Now you realize that is someone's mom, grandma, and wife, and that's not right. People would be misinformed or would misunderstand information. I heard from many members how they felt taken advantage of and preyed on. Each day was a chance for me to make a difference and hope I left the member better informed than when they started, even if it was not what they wanted to hear.

The how, when, why, and where of joining Medicare is not taught in school and people are not gathered once they turn 64 to prepare them for what is to come. So along with retirement and growing old, you now have to learn all about this government insurance coverage that you are required to have. This book is for every senior or loved one of anyone going into Medicare or already living within it. There are a thousand things to learn and it can be very frustrating to not understand it and feel it is out of your control. Keep this book handy, recommend it to those at church, people at the doctor's office, and share it with family. Help educate each other in this process.

> FACT: There are more misinformed members then informed members!

And education is what I want to do here. As a former health teacher I have found I have quite the knack for explaining things to people in a way that actually makes sense. When I decided to change from working with youth to instead working with Medicare part D seniors, it turns out the job wasn't too different. I would not call myself an expert with a certificate and degree, but pretty darn close. This book will not explain every minutia and exception to the plan. I hope to teach the basics while making it easier to understand. There are complicated ideas that are easy to get confused and make you feel defeated. I want to ease those fears and help put you back in control of your own health, time, and finances.

> *Every day I would be told "Oh bless your heart hunny," or "I rarely take advice from 'you people', but YOU have a good head on your shoulders and have given me more information than anyone, I understand now."*

There are certain things you just have to accept. Remember, this is a Medicare plan. In other words, a federal plan. There are different rules that have to be followed. Medicare will set standards and rules, and the plans can all slightly vary around those limits. But you have to accept you have to play by their rules. Just remind yourself, "It is better than paying for the whole thing myself." I absolutely understand there are constraints on your money, you cannot always choose different medications that cost less, and there are other obstacles, but at least be as informed as possible. Do yourself a favor; take notes, reread, and think about all those who aren't as fortunate to understand this Medicare frustration, *it is literally a matter of life or death*.

I will also use plenty of words to describe everything as much as possible. If you don't like that, skim the headings and check the topics to see what applies best to what you are looking for. Look for the personal stories that you may be able to directly relate to because they do come from real people. And as a teacher, I know a review and main points of a chapter is always best for those that just want to flip to the end of the chapter and check it out. Plus, if you get lost in the alphabet soup at any point, refresh yourself with the lingo listed in Chapter 10.

After reading this book you will be informed in your own health and finances to make the best choice for yourself. Your needs most likely will be much different at age 65 and at 95. Changes under our current Presidential and Congressional leadership will in all likelihood make the next round of changes to coverage and eligibility. At the current rate of spending with our aging population, there are frequent changes to Medicare, and some even go as far to estimate that Medicare may be exhausted by *2030*. So this will arm you for today…So let's get prepared and ahead of the game, let's get started!

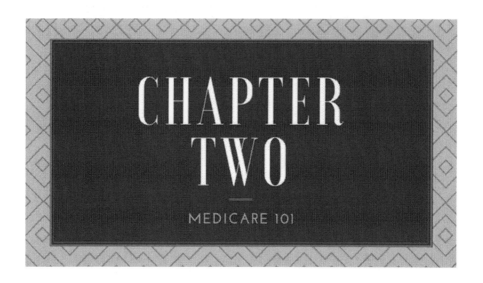

CHAPTER TWO

MEDICARE 101

Customer: "So is this Obamacare or Trump's fault?"
Me: "No, this is just Medicare." (**Thinking, it's going to be a long day)

WHAT IS MEDICARE AND WHAT HAS IT BECOME?

A Little History

Medicare started as a social insurance program designed to help the elderly and disabled get health insurance. After the Great Depression when illness ran rampant, the Social Security Act was started to provide assistance for those in need. With the Baby Boom post World War II it was obvious our population was exploding and more services would be needed in our nation. By 1965, this developed into the Social Security Act that spawned Medicare and Medicaid programs. Over the years this has been added to and subtracted from. Initially, Medicare began as just hospital coverage with the option of medical for those over 65. Then it was extended to those on disability with long term illness.

Additional services were added, oversite increased to keep prices in check, and eventually prescription drug coverage came on board.

Medicaid is different than Medicare...

Remember, MedicAID is assistance for low-income individuals or families and MediCARE is for those over 65 or with disability.

You *can* be eligible for both.

The Briefest of Overviews

A quick description of each part of Medicare is listed below along with how prescription drug coverage may fall into those categories.

PART A IS HOSPITAL INSURANCE

Part A is available to all citizens over the age of 65 that have work and paid taxes into social security for the required 40 quarters, or 10 years. This is a covered plan that does not require premiums because you have already paid for it with your taxes, that evil FICA deductions that you see taking your money from your paycheck each week. If you have not met this requirement you may still be eligible under your spouse's qualifying experience or to pay into the system. This helps to cover cost of inpatient hospital stays, skilled nursing facilities, and home health care. There are rules for what qualifies, when and how much is covered by this insurance, having to do with the length and type of stay, as well as a cap on the total amount paid out.

FACT: Other parts of Medicare may pay for hospital coverage if part A is exhausted.

PART B IS MEDICAL INSURANCE

Medicare Part B helps to cover the cost of medical services, such as doctor visits, outpatient care, home health services, some preventive care, some preventative services, and durable medical equipment such as a nebulizer, glucose meter, and wheelchairs. Participation is optional and you are eligible if you qualify for Part A. A premium is paid to Medicare and generally covers 80% of allowable charges. Additional supplemental coverage is offered through private insurance or Medigap plans.

> FACT: Organ transplants may be covered by Medicare, in which case part B continues to cover ongoing costs related to surgery, including medications.

PART C IS A COMBINATION PLAN

Medicare has approved insurance companies that have plans that offer a combination of Medicare services A, B, and D, known as Medicare Advantage. The premiums are set by the plan depending on their services offered or additional services included like vision or dental. Often times these plans may be an HMO or PPO.

PART D IS THE PRESCRIPTION DRUG INSURANCE

Part D are plans offered by Medicare approved insurance companies. Each plan has its own list of covered medications, deductibles, copay and/or coinsurance, and premiums. Participation is voluntary as long as you have prescription drug coverage as good as Medicare. Without enrollment you can be assessed a penalty by Medicare. Part D covers outpatient prescription medications, based on the rules of Part D and the prescription drug plan.

> FACT: Fees exist, it is a business like a bank

Instances medications might be covered by other parts of Medicare:

- Medications may be paid for under **Part A** if they are administered in the hospital or as a direct result of that stay, or some medications during hospice.

- Some medications or supplies may be covered under Part B for those in nursing homes or used in home health services. Medication or disposable supplies that need a prescription but go with equipment paid by **Part B** may also be covered by Part B, like test strips and lancets for diabetics and albuterol for a nebulizer. Part B may also pay for some inpatient medications after Part A resources are exhausted.
- Medication coverage can be a part of a **Part C** plan but depends on what the plan includes.

This is Medicare in a nutshell. There are times there are conflicts between the parts of the plan that may argue who has to pick up the tab or under what specific circumstance. In general, Medicare will pay out first and then coordinate any secondary insurances or benefits before you are given the remainder of the bill. Not all plans for supplemental medical, Medicare Advantage, or Prescription Drug Plan are made equal. Medicare has standards for plans that they must meet and in some cases standards that they cannot exceed. But within these ranges is where you are left to find the best coverage for yourself.

So now that you know the difference between A, B, C, and D, here is a simple way to remember...know let's get started on the basics

REVIEW

A	B	C	D
HOSPITAL	**MEDICAL**	**COMBINATION**	**DRUG PLAN**
Inpatient hospital coverage,	Outpatient medical care for doctor	Medicare Advantage Plans, outside	Prescription medication insurance,

free to most based on years worked and has a deductible	visits and health equipment, Monthly Premium for coverage	insurance covering Parts A, B, and sometimes D	required to have a plan once 65

1. If Debra needs compression socks, which Part of Medicare would pay?
2. Anthony is in the hospital for a week, who pays for coverage?
3. Margaret orders Insulin, diabetic test strips, and Atorvastatin, who pays?
4. What is included in a Medicare Advantage plan?

Answers
1. B, for medical equipment
2. A, hospital stay
3. Insulin and Atorvastatin are paid by Part D, diabetic test strips go with equipment so Part B will pay.
4. Medicare Advantage plans will have hospital and medical coverage with the some plans also including prescription drug coverage.

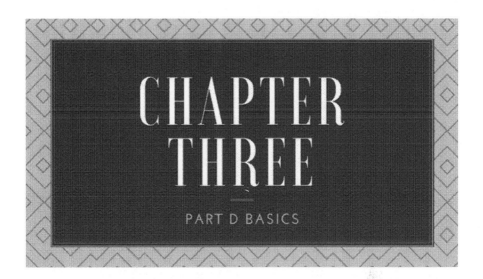

CHAPTER THREE

PART D BASICS

> *Customer: "I don't take medicine, why am I paying for this plan?"*
> *Me: "If you don't have a plan once you turn 65, the government will charge you a penalty once you do add one."*
> *(**Thinking...you obviously didn't read the large print 400 page literature that killed a rain forest to print)*

Prescription drug coverage has not always been a part of Medicare. When it was added in 2006 there were many more questions than answers for seniors trying to wade through the mountain of paperwork with, of course, the lack of helpful information. I remember watching my dad try to help my grandparents sign up. They all sat around the rotary phone (yes it's the 2000's but it is grandparents) with the application forms trying to decide if they should sign up, will the medications be covered, what will the cost be, will the doctors or pharmacist accept this. I'm sure there are a few less rotary phones today, but the questions haven't changed much for many.

> FACT: Children calling on behalf of their parents are just as, if not more, frustrated with the confusion than their parents.

Once you turn 65 and you have a Medicare Part A and/or Part B plan, you are eligible, you have to decide if you want a Medicare Rx plan or is you current coverage enough? It is not mandatory to have a Part D plan, but it is required that the plan you have is considered creditable coverage, or simply said, 'as good as Medicare's plan'. This may mean your current or previous employer's insurance coverage is sufficient to meet these standards. You can take a look at other Prescription Drug Plans but can choose to stay with your current coverage if it meets your needs.

I keep saying that Medicare has standards for insurances that are allowed to have Part D drug plans, now I'll elaborate a bit on what this means.

Part D plans are <u>individual plans</u>. This may be the first time since getting married that you and your spouse do not have joint plans. In the same way, following federal HIPAA standards, you cannot call up and give or get information on your spouse's plan just because you are married. Because this is all medical information, it is protected unless you as the member give verbal permission or have a Power of Attorney document on file with the plan. This is one of those rules you just have to accept and get used to.

> FACT: Just because they are individual plans does not mean you cannot speak about your partners plan and then ask them to switch over then look at your plan.

A <u>premium</u> threshold is set for the year. There is a minimum rate that must be offered and plans are even given incentive to be at the minimum as they can get automatic enrollees that are granted coverage due to their Medicaid coverage. Plans may have a higher premium if they offer greater services, such as higher coverage or lower copays, but this is based on business models for a money making business. The premium may be paid in full by the member, or if a part of a group coverage by employer or city group, the premium may be paid by the group.

A plan may or may not have a deductible, and it could be applied to all medications or only those on certain tier levels. This set amount has to be paid before agreed to rates (copays or coinsurance) go into effect. Don't worry, we will break this down in the next chapter.

Covered medications are documented on the plan formulary. This list of approved medications must include at least two medications from each class of drugs available by Medicare, and some medications are required to be added to the list if medically necessary. These medications do have to be prescriptions, so no over-the-counter medications, must be used and sold in the US. A plan will not be able to send you your medications overseas or pay for anything not sold or approved in the US.

Certain categories of medications, plans are required to cover a majority of drugs - not just the minimum of two per category. These would include drugs classified as

- antidepressants,
- antipsychotics,
- anticonvulsants,
- immunosuppressants,
- cancer medications, and
- HIV/AIDS treatments.

I'm going to keep it simple. Every prescription drug plan cannot offer every medication made. However this list of categories must give you a majority of the options. If you are on an antidepressant, the plan cannot offer to cover Zoloft and Prestiq while not covering any other medications. Instead they must cover the vast majority of drugs in this group, which prevents high prices to consumers and monopolies in drug companies.

There are also medications that, according to Medicare, are <u>NOT</u> approved to be covered by the plan unless they are deemed medically necessary for approved treatments. Did you know that these are not covered?

- fertility drugs,
- weight loss and gain,
- over-the-counter,
- Rx vitamins and minerals (with some exceptions),
- cough and cold relief drugs,
- sexual and erectile dysfunction,
- cosmetic,
- drugs that require monitoring services, and
- drugs unregister by manufacturers with the FDA or who don't have gap discount program agreements with Centers for Medicare and Medicaid Services (CMS)

A great example of excluded medications being APPROVED would been when Viagra or Cialis is written for enlarged prostate disease or weight gain medication after someone has had treatment for cancer or HIV.

Each plan must also have a Medicare approved <u>tier</u> structure. I will give examples of this nitty-gritty in the next chapter, but essentially this is putting each medication on the formulary into a category that copays are based on. A plan may have 2 tiers or up to 5. Each tier will have its own copay or coinsurance, and on some lucky plans they may even have some tiers without a copay.

Network Pharmacies must be dedicated to this plan. A plan will have covered network pharmacies that they will pay for claims at and could have *Preferred* pharmacies with a better rate than standard pharmacies.

REVIEW

- ★ You <u>must</u> have a prescription drug plan once you turn 65 (This is called Medicare Part D).

★ Prescription Drug Plans are <u>individual</u> plans
★ Medications listed on the <u>formulary</u> are covered by the plan.
★ A <u>deductible</u> may have to be paid before copays are offered.
★ You can <u>ask</u> a plan to cover a medication not on their approved list.
★ Medications are placed on <u>tiers</u> for pricing.

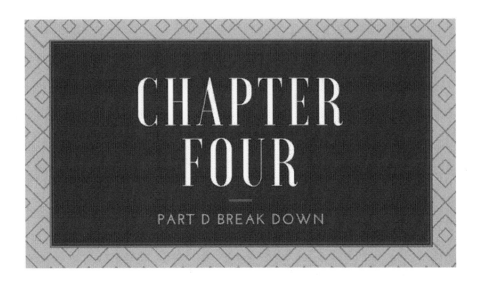

CHAPTER FOUR

PART D BREAK DOWN

Customer: "You take money from my Social Security every month, what am I paying for?"

Me: "A much lower rate than if you were to pay out of pocket, let me help you understand," (*Thinking...here we go again)

So far, Part D sounds pretty simple, much like many other insurance plans. But again, remember this is a federally approved plan within their structure and guidelines, so there is more to understand. If you do have questions, do not feel alone - you are simply thinking ahead! Hopefully I will help you with some of that here. I will talk mostly about 2018 pricing to help most people in deciphering next year's plans.

Drug Plan Structure

Each Prescription Drug Plan (PDP) has a premium which is paid in full by the member or the group that has organized the plan for them. There are exceptions with federal help, but generally speaking, this is a member's responsibility, not the plan. What you are paying for is access to more affordable care. Prices of medication may be high, but consider what they may be if you were only paying out of pocket? Prescription Drug Plans have agreements with drug manufacturers and have a negotiated lower rate that they agree to charge for the medications. When a Prescription Drug Plan is bringing thousands of members to the plate, a manufacturer will agree on a lowered rate to get this quantity of members.

Prescription Drug Plans have drug coverage phases set up by Medicare. These include the initial drug coverage phase, the coverage cap, and catastrophic phase and may or may not include a deductible. The thresholds of the three main levels of coverage rates are set by Medicare each year.

A Drug plan may choose to have a deductible or not. If they do, this is the amount you have to pay before your plan coverage goes into effect. In 2017 the deductible threshold set by Medicare that no plan could exceed was $400 and will increase only slightly for 2018 to $405. Many plans do not have a deductible or it may only apply to medications in certain tiers, usually the higher tiers and higher priced medications.

To understand the chart below, these are the Medicare standard for the three phases.

	2017	2018
Initial drug spend	$0 – 3,700	$0 - $3,750
Coverage Gap (TrOOP)	$3,701 - $4,950	$3,751 - $5,000
Catastrophic	$4,951 +	$5,001 +

Follow these charts as you work your way through the levels of coverage and remember the key terms needed for each:

The plan will keep track of money spent by each group of payers involved
- Drug Spend - total paid by you and the plan
- True Out of Pocket (TrOOP) - what you, as the member, have paid
- Plan Spend - what the plan has spent
- Medicare Spend - portion Medicare pays while you are in the coverage gap or catastrophic phase
- Other payers - secondary insurances or programs that also pay toward prescription costs

PHASE 1, INITIAL COVERAGE

The Initial Coverage phase begins January 1st each year, or the start date of when your plan begins. If you have a deductible, initial coverage will begin once the deductible has been met. How long you remain in the initial phase is based on the Total Drug Spend for your plan. This means what both you AND the plan pays together. If you have a medication with a $10 copay, but the plan pays the remaining $27 of the cost of the medication, then the drug spend is $37. This will be added up until you reach a total of $3,750 in 2018. Anything you have paid toward the deductible will also go toward this total.

FACT: Many customers don't realize that one medication can put them into the coverage gap

PHASE 2, COVERAGE GAP

The dreaded Coverage Gap often times goes by the much sweeter-than-it-really-is name of the "donut hole". This is when you have a "gap or hole" in coverage. Previous to the Affordable Care Act

(ACA), this was a large gap in coverage when members had to pay 100% of the cost of medication! The ACA worked to gradually close that gap. The plan was to take a 10 year period, between 2010 and 2020 and gradually increase the percent that drug plans pay, while decreasing the amount that members pay. For drug manufacturers to be allowed to be a part of Medicare Part D, they also have to agree to pay 50% of the price of brand medications while members are in the Gap. So once you and the plan have spent $3,750 on your medications, you are now in 2018 are required to pay 44% of the cost of generic medications, and 35% of brand.

FACT: Good news, if your monthly average drug spend in 2018 is under $312, you will not reach the gap!

Getting into the coverage gap is often seen as a horrible event. You may have had a $40 copay for your inhaler in the initial coverage and it has now gone to $250...but remember, just 8 years ago you would have been paying the full cost of that medication which would have been $625, instead of just the 40% share. Just know you aren't alone if you are in this gap or will be entering this section. There are resources included in Chapter 12

FACT: If your medications are more than $702 a month you will get out of the Coverage Gap!

PHASE 3, CATASTROPHIC COVERAGE

While being in the coverage gap is horrible, being in the Catastrophic is actually good! Once your Total Out of Pocket cost, meaning what you alone have paid toward your medications this year (does NOT include your monthly premiums), reaches the amount of $5,000, you leave the coverage gap and head into catastrophic coverage. You now pay a much lower price, but of course this takes a little explaining too...

- Brands - pay 5% cost of medication or $8.35, whichever is greater
- Generics - pay 5% cost of medication or $3.35, whichever is greater

That same brand name inhaler from the coverage gap now costs $31.25!

Now that you understand the phases of one year in a Prescription Drug Plan, now let's discuss tier structure...

Tier Structure

Each plan is required to have a tier structure for medications, listing how copays or coinsurance will be applied to medications on each level. Plans can have between 2 and 5 tiers, I will give a few examples to break this down.

A 2 tier plan may look like this:
- Tier 1 - Preferred Generics
- Tier 2 - Non-Preferred generics and brands

A 5 tier plan may look like this:
- Tier 1 - Preferred Generics - lowest cost medications, some plans don't have any cost for this tier
- Tier 2 - Non preferred generics and preferred brands
- Tier 3 - Non-preferred brands
- Tier 4 - High-priced or specialty
- Tier 5 - Specialty

All plans are different so it is important to pay attention to the tiers structure, how they are covered, and what each plan includes.

> FACT: Medications can fall on different tiers on different plans.
> Different tiers = different prices

Generally generic medications are less expensive, however that does not mean they are always in the lowest tiers or lower prices. High priced medications and new generics may still fall into a higher tier until there is enough competition in the market to bring prices down.

Some plans may have a deductible for some tiers, all tiers, or none at all.

To better explain this, a few examples of plans and copays:

	Plan A $250 Deductible tiers 3-5 No Gap Coverage Premium - $40/month	Plan B No Deductible Tiers 1 & 2 Copay in CovGap Premium - $120/month	Plan C No Deductible No Gap Coverage Premium - $95/month
Tier 1	$5	$5	$10
Tier 2	$15	$10	$20
Tier 3	$35	$20	$60
Tier 4	40%	$50	---
Tier 5	22%	25%	---

The premium is a set rate that will remain the same each month for the whole plan year and will not change or go toward your drug price accumulations.

PRACTICE: Follow these examples and check to see if you understand the copay and coinsurance amounts. *Remember, coinsurance is when you pay a percent of the price of the medication instead of a set amount for a copay, like shown in Tier 5 and on Plan A in Tier 4. If a $100 medication is a Tier 4 on A, the coinsurance would be $40.

COST OF DRUG, INITIAL PHASE

Example 1: Levothyroxine, Cost of medication (drug spend) $60 (example how drugs can fall under different tiers in different plans)

- Plan A - Tier 2 = **$15** copay
- Plan B - Tier 1 = **$5** copay
- Plan C - Tier 1 = **$10** copay

Example 2: Ventolin Inhaler, Cost of medication $700
- Plan A - Tier 3 = $250 (if deductible not met) + $35 copay = **$285**
- Plan B - Tier 3 = **$20** copay
- Plan C - Tier 3 = **$60** copay

Example 3: Humira *Specialty Rx*, Cost of medication $2,000
- Plan A - Tier 5 = $2,000 x 22% = **$444** coinsurance
- Plan B - Tier 5 = $2,000 x 25% = **$500** coinsurance
- Plan C - Tier 3 = **$60** copay

COST OF DRUG, COVERAGE GAP PHASE

Now that your plan is in the coverage gap, this chart shows what copays and coinsurance will look like on those same three plans. Remember, Plan B covers the Gap in tiers 1 & 2, so medications will stay with the same copay.

	Plan A	Plan B	Plan C

	$250 Deductible tiers 3-5 No Gap Coverage Premium - $40/month	No Deductible Tiers 1 & 2 Copay in CovGap Premium - $120/month	No Deductible No Gap Coverage Premium - $95/month
Tier 1	40%	$5	40%
Tier 2	40%	$10	40%
Tier 3	40%	40%	40%
Tier 4	40%	40%	---
Tier 5	40%	40%	---

Example 1: Levothyroxine, Cost of medication $60
- Plan A - Tier 2 = $60 x 40% = **$24** coinsurance
- Plan B - Tier 1 = **$5** copay
- Plan C - Tier 1 = $60 x 40% = **$24** coinsurance

*Notice, Plan B allows for tiers 1 and 2 to remain copays while in the Gap

Example 2: Humira, Cost of medication $2,000
- Plan A - Tier 5 = x 40% = **$800** coinsurance
- Plan B - Tier 5 = x 40% = **$800** coinsurance
- Plan C - Tier 3 = x 40% = **$800** coinsurance

Does this help? Look at your medications, what tier do they fall into, and what phase of coverage you are in to determine the price of your medications each time you have them filled.

I would spend hours on the phone with members explaining the price of their medications, how it is different this month for the last time they picked up their medication, because of their change in phases of the plan. Understanding the Coverage Gap and Catastrophic coverages can be extremely difficult, especially if you do not understand the principles of it.

So an example...I will give an example of what could be paid on a plan using mail order as you work your way through the plan for a year.

YEAR PLAN COVERAGE EXAMPLE:

This is an example of one year of coverage through a Prescription Drug Plan.

You have plan A:

	Plan A $250 Deductible tiers 3-5 No Gap Coverage Premium - $40/month
Tier 1	$5
Tier 2	$15
Tier 3	$35
Tier 4	40%
Tier 5	22%

Your Medications:
- Omeprazole - Tier 1
- Warfarin - Tier 2
- Sensipar - Tier 3

January – You have each prescription filled as a 90 day fill

I have compiled a basic chart to show the cost of the medications and who pays each portion.

	Member	Plan	Total (Drug Spend)
Omeprazole	$4	$0	$4
Warfarin	$15	$2	$17
Sensipar	$285	$1,315	$1,600
Total	**$304 + $40 premium**	**$1,317**	**$1,621**

- Omeprazole - you pay the full price of the medication because the price is less than the copay ($5) for a tier 1 medication.
- Warfarin - you pay the copay and the plan pays the remained.
- Sensipar - deductible for the plan needs to be met. Pay out of pocket the first $250 to meet the deductible, then pay the copay ($35) for the remainder of your share to cover the medication this fill, plan pays the remainder.
- **Your bill for January will be $344 (medications and premium)**
- Total Drug Spend is $1,612 (watching to know when we will go into the Gap)

February – Your bill for February will be **$40 (premium)**

March – Your bill for March will be **$40 (premium)**

April – You have each prescription refilled as a 90 day fill

	Member	Plan	Total (Drug Spend)
Omeprazole	$4	$0	$4
Warfarin	$15	$2	$17
Sensipar	$35	$1,565	$1,600
Total	**$54 + $40 premium**	**$1,567**	**$1,621**

- Omeprazole - you pay the full price of the medication because the price is less than the copay for a tier 1 medication.
- Warfarin - you pay the copay and the plan pays the remained.
- Sensipar - deductible has been met. Pay copay for tier 3 medication and the plan pays the remainder
- **Your bill for April will be $94 (medications and premium)**
- Total Drug Spend is $3,242 (watching to know when we will go into the <u>Gap</u>)

Pop Quiz

Do you remember what the amount is for Drug Spend to push you into the Coverage Gap?

****Answer: $3,750

May – Your bill for May will be **$40 (premium)**

June – Your bill for June will be **$40 (premium)**

July – You have each prescription refilled as a 90 day fill

	Member	Plan (and Manufacturer)	Total (Drug Spend)
Omeprazole	$4	$0	$4
Warfarin	$15	$2	$17
Sensipar	?	?	?
Total			

THIS is the month you will go into the coverage gap. So slowly…

Your drug spend, what has been paid in total for medications this year is $3,242.

You just had two medications filled with a full price of **$21**, bringing your drug spend to **$3,263**.

You will reach the Coverage Gap when your drug spend hits **$3,750**.

This is in **$508**.

So for Sensipar, the first $508 of the cost of the medication you will pay the **$35 copay** because you are still in the Initial Coverage.

Let's do the break down.
- Sensipar costs $1600
- You paid the copay to complete the remaining $508 of the initial coverage
- This leaves the remaining drug cost of **$1,092.**
  - $1,600 – $ 508 = $1,092
- Now you are in the Coverage Gap and will pay 40% of the $1,092

- o $1,092 x 40% = **$436.80**
- $35 copay + $436.80 coinsurance from coverage gap = **$471.80**

Remainder of July's chart:

Sensipar	**$471.80**	$1,128.20	$1,600
Total	**490.80 + $40 premium**	**$1,130.20**	**$1,621**

***For <u>brand</u> medications in the coverage gap, the manufacturer covers 50% of the drug spend, **$556.50**.

- **Your bill for July will be $530.80 (medications and premium)**
  - $471.80 + $21 = $490.80 (Omeprazole, Warfarin, Senispar)
  - $490.80 + $40 premium = $530.80

Your Out-Of-Pocket Cost is $848.80 (watching to know when we will go into <u>Catastrophic</u> coverage)
- Out-Of-Pocket figured by adding price you have paid for <u>medications</u> so far this year
  - o January $304
  - o February $0
  - o March $0
  - o April $54
  - o May $0
  - o June $0
  - o July $490.80
  - o Year to date total-out-of-pocket = $848.80

August – Your bill for August will be **$40 (premium)**

September - Your bill for September will be **$40 (premium)**

October – You have each prescription refilled as a 90 day fill

Pop Quiz

Why are the numbers on this chart different?

***Answer: You are in the Coverage Gap and will pay 40% of the Drug Spend:

	Member	Plan (and Manufacturer)	Total (Drug Spend)
Omeprazole	$1	$3	$4
Warfarin	$6.80	$10.20	$17
Sensipar	$640	$960	$1600
Total	**$647.80 + $40 premium**	**$973.20**	**$1621**

***For <u>brand</u> medications in the coverage gap, the manufacturer covers 50% of the drug spend, **$800**.

- **Your bill for October will be $687.80 (medications and premium)**
- Your Out-Of-Pocket Cost is $1496.60 (watching to know when we will go into <u>Catastrophic</u> coverage)
    - Prior months total-out-of pocket = $848.80 (see July's breakdown)
    - August $0
    - September $0
    - October $647.80

November - Your bill for August will be **$40 (premium)**

December - Your bill for August will be **$40 (premium)**

Total Cost Spent for 2018:

	Member	Plan
Premium	$40 x 12months = **$480**	$0
Medication Cost	**$1,496.60**	$4,987.40

You ended the year in the <u>Coverage Gap</u>.

You did not reach <u>Catastrophic</u> because what you paid out of pocket for medications did not exceed $5000.

January 2019 all accumulated amounts will reset to $0. Deductible will start over and you will begin in the Initial Coverage Phase.

Before the new year starts, you want to check for any changes to the plan, for example:
- Will the deductible change?
- Will my medications change tiers or no longer be covered?
- Will new alternatives or generics be available?
- Does this plan still best fit my needs?

REVIEW

- ★ What you are paying for when joining the plan is a reduced rate for medications that your insurance (this prescription drug plan) is paying a shared part of.
- ★ Phase of Prescription Drug Plan
  - ○ Deductible (if applicable)
  - ○ Initial
  - ○ Coverage Gap
  - ○ Catastrophic

★ You can stay in one phase of the plan all year, one medication can put you through all of the phases at once, or anywhere in between.
★ Pay attention to not just what you pay out of pocket for medications, but also the Total Drug Spend, since this is what can put you into the Coverage Gap.

In the next chapter we will look at all the hands in the cookie jar of you Prescription Drug Plan.

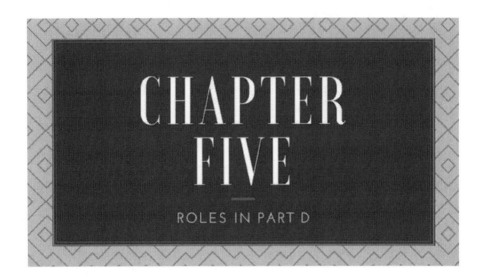

CHAPTER FIVE

ROLES IN PART D

Customer: "Who is responsible for this mess? It must be you people!"
Me: (**Sigh, oh good 'you people') "Well let me see how I can help you ma'am"

The main answer needs to be YOU! Your health will be of Number One importance to you, anyone else involved is going to have more than just you to consider. Keep records, double check others in the circle, and know who the correct person is to contact for results.

Let's get real. On the surface you think there is only you, the doctor, and pharmacists involved in you getting your prescriptions. In reality there is everyone involved in Medicare, insurance, and computer that never seem to get it right.

So, let's talk about a few of the people and their roles that hidden in the shadows playing a very hands on role in your medication process:

Doctor

- Only person who writes Prescription
- Can approve alternative medications

Nurse/Assistant

- Sends prescription to pharmacy
- Can call drug coverage customer service for you

After Hours Service

- Many offices provide on-call doctors for emergencies
- May be able to prescribe short-term prescriptions

Pharmacist

- Responsible for drugs given to you
- Can recommend alternatve or generic drugs to help lower cost

Pharmacist Tech

- Can help you with running drugs through Medicare B or D
- Able to transfer your prescription to another pharmacy or mail order

Local Pharmacy

- May have a higher cost than mail order
- Works one on one with you

Prescription Drug Insurance Provider

- Has mulitple departments, know which one you need

Customer Service Representative

- Assist with plan, billing, enrollment, coverage, and exceptions
- If combined with Mail Order Pharmacy, may also assist in ordering medications

Exception Board

- Supervisors make decisions on return of drugs and disputes over payments
- Approve formulary exceptions

Medicare System

- Broken down into main Parts A, B, & D
- Know which one you need

Medicare A & B

- Customer service representatives within both systems
- One incident may cover multiple Parts of Medicare

Broker

- They sell you the plan you desire
- They may make a commision on the sale
- Must be certified to sell insurance to you

Member (you)

- Responisble for all your drug needs
- Works with doctor, customer service, and pharmacist

Power of Attorney

- Documentation needs to be on file with Doctor, Drug plan, and pharmacy
- Can make decisions on behalf of member

Child or Partner of Member

- Member needs to give permission for access to accounts
- May call drug plan on their behalf, but in order to refill scripts the member must give approval

FACT: Customer Care for the Prescription Drug Plan and mail order pharmacy would not exist if the process ran smoothly

As you can tell from prior chapters you, the sales broker, the customer service representative, have built a foundation. In the next chapters we will discover the importance of the other roles.

CHAPTER SIX

COMMON ISSUES

> Customer: *"I guess I'll just die then."*
> Me: *"Oh no sir, no one wants that, let me see what I can do for you"* (**Thinking, I hope he listens!)

Here is where I share the horror stories, common complaints, and complications...

Q: *"My doctor prescribed this medicine, how dare you tell me I can't have it. Are you calling my doctor stupid? Are you saying he's wrong?"*

A: No. There are many reasons a medication may not be immediately covered by the plan:
- It may not be on the list of covered medications = request a <u>formulary exception</u>
- It may be on list of covered medications but may need additional information before it can be granted based on medication use of safety = complete a '<u>prior authorization</u>'

- The dose may exceed what the plan allows = request a quantity limit exception

Doctors also have patients on countless drug plans, they do not know what is covered on each plan or what may be less expensive.
- Ask a pharmacist or nurse to check your formulary to see if a generic is covered by the plan or an alternative medication that may be used for the same purposes.

Q: "I am going on vacation but will run out of medication while I'm gone."

A: Check with your plan, they may allow you to get prescriptions filled early. They can place an override in the system to fill your prescription sooner than they would normally allow. Each plan is different, so be sure you check all the policies and rules before you assume this will be allowed. You may have to have your medications delivered to you or filled at another location if you are vacationing in the United States, or if out of the country you may have them sent to a friend or relative that can forward them on to you.

Other possible reasons for overrides that you may be able to get an early or extra release of medication:
- Lost medication
- Mail order lost before delivery
- Change in doctors directions to increase usage

Using your medications incorrectly is NOT a reason for an override! You may have to pay out of pocket or speak to your doctor to get medication.

Check with you plan, not all overrides may be options and there may be limits, such as only one use per year.

Q: "My medication costs how much?! Well then I guess I just won't take it. You just want me to die!"

A: Prices of medications are set by manufacturers and a negotiated lowered rate is charged by your Prescription Drug Plan. However, these prices can be astronomical. I will talk about this more thoroughly in Chapter 8 on saving money, but a common option that most do not know about is a tiering exception. You can question your plan and ask to have your medication covered at a lower tier level. If a similar medication is covered at that lower level but there is a legitimate reason why you have to be on this higher priced medication it may be granted. That's right, you ask to pay less! Make a request with the Coverage Determination Department of your prescription drug plan and their Exception Board will decide if that tier can be lowered.

Q: "I asked you to cover my medication and you denied it, why?!"

A: Not all exception requests are granted, there are qualifications that must be met for it to be granted and it is reviewed by an advisory panel. However, a denial does not mean you are now out of luck, there is a thorough process.

1. Ask for an exception (formulary, tiering, prior authorization, etc)
   a. If denied...
2. Ask for an appeal, the prescription drug plan will reconsider and let you know if initial needed information was not received
   a. If denied...
3. Request a redetermination from an outside independent group. The Prescription Drug Plan will provide information on an outside party that considers appeals
   a. If denied....
4. Appeal hearing with an Administrative Law Judge

a. If denied…
5. Request a review by the Medicare Appeals Council
    a. If denied…
6. Request a Federal district court judicial review

FACT: Sometimes asking a Customer Service Representative for their opinion may lead you down a path that you did not know you had before. Don't be afraid to ask, they have resources!

Q: "My doctor said I needed a shingles vaccine, will you pay for it?"

A: Some vaccines can be covered by Medicare part D, often times including shingles, tetanus, and pneumonia. However, Medicare rules to this as well:
- Covered vaccines will be listed on your formulary, see what is approved.
- A doctor's office may be considered "out of network"
    - Go to a pharmacy to get a vaccine from "in network"
    - This is not a clinic in the pharmacy!
- The doctor's office may run the claim through part B, ask them to switch to run it through part D.
- There may also be a fee for the administration of the vaccine that is not covered by the prescription drug pan and you will pay for out of pocket.
- Vaccines are often a higher tier. This could be the only medication you have that falls into deductible, so you may pay full price out of pocket if the deductible has not been met.
- File a claim if the vaccine is not paid for at first. You can submit your information to the plan and if covered receive reimbursement.

Q: "My husband died, I need to disenroll him from the plan."

A: Funeral homes will submit death certificates to Social Security, who will notify Medicare, and this will disenroll members from the plan. You may contact the plan to make them aware, but Medicare will make the official disenrollment.

Deaths are also difficult because Power of Attorney on an account is no longer effective. Customer Service should be able to assist with being sure phone acknowledgements are turned off and auto-refill discontinued, but this is about the extent of what can be handled without documentation of an Executor of Estate on file.

Also check with the plan on their policy with returns. If a medication has not been opened, it may be refundable. Premiums for the plan are owed for the current month of death, any overpayments will be returned.

REVIEW

★ Know which phase of the drug plan you are in and how close you are to moving into the next phase.
★ Don't be afraid to ask questions – know the full cost of your medications, what tier you are in, and options if you do run into an issue
★ Do your research before you pay – see you have options to pay less or have other medications covered by the plan
★ Have a plan for your family in case of your death

CHAPTER SEVEN

COMMON SENSE

Customer: *"I know my doctor is closed for the weekend, that's why I'm calling you."*
Me: *(**Thinking, Oh geez, is this a prank. Let's see what we can do for you since you took your last pill this morning but didn't call until 7pm on a Friday!!!!)*

Think of when businesses are open and when they are closed, and how long things take when relying on more than one person. You know your doctor can call in a prescription to the pharmacy and it can be ready in an hour, but that is under the best of circumstances. I am not trying to make anyone feel bad or not want to reach out when they need medicine. Everyone is forgetful and this can increase with age, but these mistakes are not what I am talking about. I will be the first to understand forgetting to do something important like this; do not hesitate to call and ask for help solving this problem! However, we do try to help set you up to avoid these situations and everyone needs habits to have the best situation. So use common sense, for example: DON'T BE A BETTY...

A doctor has to <u>write</u> you a prescription.	"No Betty, you can't just ask for a prescription at the pharmacy."
A doctor has to <u>send</u> the prescription to a pharmacy, and written the <u>correct</u> way.	"Betty, You cannot just tell me how you want this filled."
If the doctor <u>changes</u> the directions how you should take the medication, it needs to be written on a new prescription	"Yes Betty, the doctor may have told you to take 2 a day now, but I cannot give you double until that is written in a prescription."
If the pharmacy is <u>busy</u>, they may not be able to fill the prescription right away.	"I'm sorry Betty, we will not have that ready until tomorrow."
If you are using a mail order pharmacy, you have to consider <u>processing and shipping</u> time.	"No Ms Betty, we cannot have this medicine you are ordering now in your mailbox tomorrow morning."
If you are <u>late</u> ordering your medicine you may not get it in time.	"Betty, you forgot to order your medicine, you may have to wait a few days or pay more for delivery or for your local pharmacy."
If you have a prescription filled at the local pharmacy you will have to wait for mail order, and vice versa.	"Insurance requires you use two-thirds of your medication Betty, you can't get another 90 days here when you just ordered that same amount from mail order yesterday."

If you are out of medication, you cannot expect to get it immediately unless you have an active prescription with refills remaining on file.

For mail order, don't yell at them because it is Friday and your medication won't process and ship until Monday. Call sooner!

If there is a holiday coming up, consider what will be open and what will be closed for these days. Same applies to the mail service.

A Prescription Drug Plan is drug insurance. They will tell you a percent must be used before you can get the next fill, generally around 70% used.
- 30 day prescription, must wait about 20 days before next fill
- 90 day prescription, must wait around 60 days before next fill
- 7 day prescription, must wait 5-6 days before next fill
- Sooo...if you want to order mail order but pick up a week's supply at the local pharmacy, mail order will not be able to process the new order until you have only 1 or 2 days remaining
- Controlled substances or specialty medications may have a longer wait time and shorter window to get refills.

<u>Read the information you get from your plan!</u>

Medicare is required to provide you with certain information, and even though you may often feel flooded with information or that you have cost an entire forest its life, there is good information in here. Two main documents:
- Explanation Of Benefits (EOB) - understand how your money is spent and where you are in your coverage. Each month you have had an active claim on your account you will receive this statement. It will show:
  - What you paid for medications,
  - What the plan paid for those medications,
  - What your total drug spend and total out of pocket cost has been for the year, which tells you...
  - What level of drug coverage you are in and how close you are to the next level.

- Annual Notice Of Change (ANOC) - Each September Prescription Drug Plans notify you of what is changing in the plan for the upcoming year.
  - Are your medications going to be on the formulary next year,
  - will they change tiers,
  - is the premium and deductible to be the same?

> FACT: Most people do not read these plans and then call me and ask the exact questions that these pamphlets answer!

Address on File

If you move or are a snowbird with more than one address, update according to your plans. If medications get sent to the wrong address or you miss your bill, this is not at the fault of the drug plan. You may have to pay for your medication again or completely out of pocket because the insurance will not pay for it again for another 60 days. If you do not pay your bill you will be disenrolled and be without coverage until a time comes to enroll again. If you forget to pay March and April's premiums, and are disenrolled in May, you may not be able to get coverage again until open enrollment. This means coverage will begin January 1st and Medicare will also charge you that Late Enrollment Penalty for the 7 months you did not have coverage. Most plans will be available to call in to make these changes or even do so online.

Payment on File

If your credit card company sends you a new credit card, even if it is just a new expiration date, this needs to be updated. This may prevent you from getting your medications on time or your premium not being paid and getting disenrolled. Many people forget this and it causes delays in getting your medicine, possible disenrollment from the plan, and lots of headaches and frustration.

REVIEW
- ★ Don't be a Betty
- ★ Understand the mail order system
- ★ Update your address and credit card to avoid issues
- ★ Do not expect to get things done when offices are closed

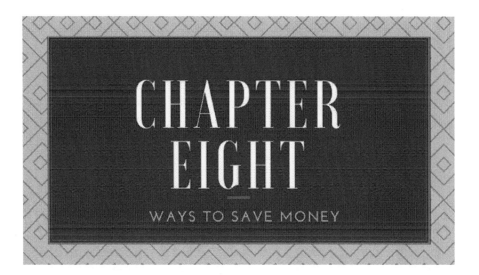

CHAPTER EIGHT

WAYS TO SAVE MONEY

> Customer: "Thank you sweetie, you just saved me so much money."
> ME; "Just doing my job (**Thinking, I am so glad you DID listen!)

This is my favorite part! This is why I wrote this book! I love finding ways for people to save money. It really is up to you to be aware of your plan, coverage, and rights. Here are some resources for saving money as well as extra tips and tricks I have picked up along the way.

Brand vs Generic vs Alternative

This is the same as shopping for any other item that could have a generic or similar product offered for sale. If you visit Costco to purchase vodka for a party, you can buy the brand, a generic, or an alternative:

- Brand - Grey Goose vodka $40
- Generic - Kirkland vodka (that is the same as Grey Goose, only without the brand name label) $20

- Alternative - Skye vodka $30

This seems simple and like it should have been in the common sense sections, but some people never think about the possibility that a very similar medication may be available for a completely different price. No changes can be made to your prescription without permission of your doctor, so collect your best information and have a talk with them.

- A <u>brand</u> medication is priced high because the manufacturer has paid to develop and test the medication. Patents last 20 years but by the time prescription hits market, the manufacturer may have less time of exclusivity
- <u>Generics</u> can use patented medication without the cost of development and testing. May initially start at a high cost but usually come down
- <u>Alternative</u> are different medications but in the same class. If they are used for the same medical purpose they may be used instead, according to doctor's discretion based on member's therapy

---

FACT: Some drug plans have savings if you use their preferred pharmacies.

Local Pharmacies

Some local pharmacies have their own savings plan. It can cost less to pay for your medications out of pocket at times. Walmart has their $4 list, GoodRx.com gives alternative savings, and so on. Just remember anything that you pay for out of pocket because it is cheaper that way, will not go toward your drug spend and accumulations on your drug plan.

Example: Levothyroxine
- Prescription Drug Plan copay: $15 copay for 30 days
- Walmart savings list: $4 for 30 days
- GoodRx coupon: $20 for 6 month

These savings are out there! It does not mean you do not need a drug plan. It just means that at times you may be able to think outside the box and in turn help yourself. If you get more savings paying out of pocket, consider that option.

Mail Order vs Local Pharmacy

A mail order pharmacy can often provide a 90 day supply at a savings, because manufacturers negotiate a rate with mail order pharmacies because of the large quantity of medication that is ordered. This can be as simple as paying one copay for a 90 day supply instead of three copays.

Example:
- Local pharmacy 30 day supply of Atorvastatin - $3
- Local pharmacy 60 day supply of Atorvastatin - $6
- Local pharmacy 90 day supply of Atorvastatin - $9
- Mail order pharmacy 30 day supply of Atorvastatin - $3
- Mail order pharmacy 90 day supply of Atorvastatin - $3

Some plans even offer lower tier medications through mail order at NO out of pocket cost or a Maximum out of Pocket (MOOP) that the plan will not allow you to exceed, they pick up the cost after this amount has been met!

Example:
- A Prescription Drug Plan with a MOOP of $500, once you have paid out of pocket for medications totally this amount, the plan will pay any expenses for medications going forward for the remainder of the calendar year.

Manufacturers

Manufacturers may be able to get you savings as well. Pay close attention to these programs, again if it is not run through the plan, the accumulators are not applying to the plan either. Did you know you can call the manufacturer and ask for a discount or find links on their website?

Social Security Extra Help

Apply with Social Security Extra Help, also known as Low Income Subsidy. If approved this can lower your monthly premium and drug costs, as well as eliminate the coverage gap. This is based on certain financial criteria and you status is reassessed each year. Do not forget to reapply each year to be sure you do not lose coverage.

> FACT: Many people are not aware of these savings...but it was right there in your Medicare enrollment. Don't be too proud to call and ask for help

State Assistance

Individual states have their own assistance plans and counselors. You may check with your local Medicare office or search online for prescription assistance. This may be a supplemental plan that is purchased or that has financial requirements to be eligible for. Each plan is different but many help to cover the costs of medication while you are in the coverage gap.

File a Claim

If you paid for something out of pocket because insurance was not on file, or applied correctly, a coverage determination was later made, or preferred network pharmacy was not available, seek reimbursement for these costs.

Your Health

This may seem like common sense or something that is completely out of your control, but is the truest statement of this book. Talk with your doctor and take responsibility for your own health and decisions. While many medications are a result of genetics, disease, and aging, a large percent are influenced by our lifestyles. Paying attention to obesity, type 2 diabetes, weight and smoking related asthma, diet, exercise, and preventative health care visits.

> FACT: The most common phone calls with complaints of the price of medications fall into two categories - INHALERS AND INSULIN

ADVICE I WOULD GIVE MY MOM!

Look at where you are in your drug coverage versus the time of year on the calendar:

Are you close to the coverage gap toward the end of the year? Consider only getting the month supply that you need instead of a 90 day supply. If this keeps you from going into the gap, let the math work for you.

Are you in catastrophic coverage? Get as many fills as possible during this year before you head back through the whole coverage cycle next year. This means possibly filling your medications as frequently as possible (every two months instead of 3). Then you will have a stash of meds to use at the beginning of next year to slow your drug spend at the start of the year.

Same goes for anyone who has a deductible. In December, see if there are any medications you can fill with your deductible met before you have to pay it again after January first.

Just the opposite goes for starting a medication that will pay toward the deductible. If your doctor gives you a new prescription in December for a medication you are paying toward the deductible for, only get a one month supply or even see if the doctor can supply you with samples until the new year. If you pay the deductible in December, you will still have to pay toward it again next year.

Do you know someone who talks about the cost of the coverage gap? This information can help them.

REVIEW

- ★ Consider generic or alternative medications
- ★ Compare savings at mail order or local pharmacies
- ★ Consider paying out of pocket for significant savings in some instances at local pharmacies
- ★ Ask for a tiering exception to lower the cost
- ★ Apply for Social Security Extra Help and look into state assistance programs
- ★ Consider where you are in the coverage year and the coverage phases

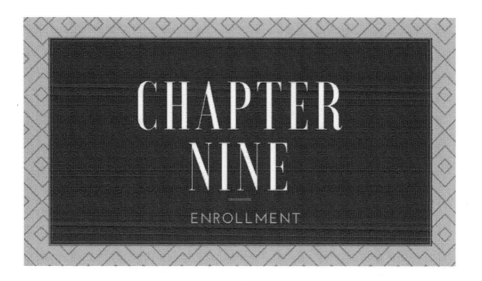

CHAPTER NINE

ENROLLMENT

> Customer: "So, are you making money when I sign up?"
> Me: "No, ma'am." (**Thinking, I wish!) "I'm not, but a broker that recommended a specific plan might get paid."

You would think the enrollment chapter would be at the start of the book as it is the start of your coverage, however I firmly believe that all of the previous information is necessary to make the best choices for your coverage.

Now that we have come full circle you have the tools to evaluate plans and compare them to your needs to make the selection that is best for you!

<u>WHEN</u> TO ENROLL
Enrollment Periods
1. <u>Initial Enrollment Period</u> -
   ○ 65 birthday - Month of birth, 3 months before, 3 months after
      ■ Example: Turn 65 on September 15th
         • Enroll June, July, August for September 1 start date

- Enroll September for October 1 start date
- Enroll October, November, December to start the first of the following month
- January first you are now out of you eligible Initial Enrollment Period

○ Disability - 25th month of disability is considered eligible for Medicare coverage, with 3 months before and after month eligible to enroll
  ■ Example: On disability for 25 months as of September
    - Enroll June, July, August for September 1 start date
    - Enroll September for October 1 start date
    - Enroll October, November, December to start the first of the following month
    - January first you are now out of you eligible Initial Enrollment Period

○ Specific severe disability that is time sensitive - immediate enrollment
  ■ Example, End Stage Renal Failure or ALS (Lou Gehrig's Disease)

2. Special Enrollment Period (SEP) - A valid reason to enroll at alternate time of the year:
○ Lose creditable coverage, retiring or employer coverage change
○ Involuntary loss of coverage
○ Move out of area or back into US
○ Move out of nursing home
○ Release from incarceration
○ Enrolled in Medicare Advantage in the last year
○ Low Income Subsidy (LIS), monthly or if status changes
○ Program of the All-Inclusive Care of the Elderly (PACE) member change
○ State Pharmaceutical Assistance Program member change
○ Enrolled during Part B General Enrollment Period: SEP April 1 - June 30
○ Medicare Advantage Disenrollment Period: SEP January 1 - February 14

- 5-star plan: SEP December 8 - November 30

3. <u>Annual Enrollment Period</u> - October 15 to December 7, for upcoming January 1 start date

If you have creditable coverage, you do not need to enroll in a new plan unless you are losing coverage.

If you have a period of time more than 63 days without coverage by a part D plan you will have a <u>Late Enrollment Penalty</u> (LEP) added to your monthly premium by Medicare.

> FACT: This LEP continues for life. The only time an LEP can be removed is if you have Medicare coverage prior to the age of 65, when you reach your 65th birthday this can be voided.

<u>Possible Additional Fees</u>: Income Related Monthly Adjustment Amount (IRMAA) - Social Security will notify you if an additional amount is owed on top of your premium due to earning a high income, $85,000 for individuals or $170,000 for joint tax filings. This is collected directly by social security and paid to the government, not the Plan.

Disenrollment is not an option whenever wanted, you must have valid disenrollment period. Just as with enrollment periods, these include life events such as moving out of area, moving into or out of a nursing home, a change in Low Income Status, and so on. You can request to disenroll from a plan, Medicare will determine you have an applicable disenrollment period or you must wait until one becomes available, such as during the annual enrollment period. To request disenrollment you may contact your plan or Medicare directly to submit through written or verbal statements.

WHY WOULD YOU BE ENROLLING IN A PRESCRIPTION DRUG PLAN

1. It is you Initial Enrollment Period: You just became eligible to enroll for the first time by turning 65 or meeting disability requirements.

2. Annual Enrollment Period: The Annual Notice of Change will be released from your current plan around September, and you can check for any formulary, copay, and premium changes to your current plan. Read over it carefully and look up each of your medications to see if the coverage will change. If you decide this is no longer the best coverage for you, now is the time that you can do something about it.

FACT: You have the option each year to change your plan

On the same note, if your health and prescription needs have changed in the last year, this is also your opportunity to change plans for more or less coverage.

3. Other qualifying Special Election Periods:
    ***If you do not have a qualifying SEP that allows you to enroll in a new plan, see if there is a 5 star plan in your Medicare region. You are allowed to switch to any 5 star plan once a year at your choosing

WHAT DO YOU NEED TO ENROLL

Have your Medicare ID card and be the enrolling member or someone that has the legal authority to speak on the member's behalf, such as power of attorney.

That's it! Just your Medicare ID card!

FACT: Enrollment only takes less than 30 minutes over the phone. Even less time when completed online, but be sure to read all disclaimers, they are the most important parts!

HOW TO ENROLL

Signing up for a part D plan is very simple and you do have a few options.

1. Enroll online at Medicare.gov or the Prescription Drug website
2. Complete a paper application and mail or fax to the plan or Medicare
3. Call the plan or Medicare and complete enrollment over the phone

Another option you are given when enrolling in the plan is that you can request your premium be deducted from your Social Security or Railroad Retirement Board benefits. You can also set his up at a later time once your plan is effective if you want to change your form of payment.

COMPARING PLANS

When comparing plans, what do you need to consider?

Start with a list of your medications. Complete this chart for each plan you want to consider:

Medications	Covered	Tier	Copay

Look at all of the elements of the plan. Some things to consider:

	YES	NO
What is the premium?	Monthly _____ For the year x 12 _____	
Is there a deductible?		
→ If so, what tiers → and amount	_____ _____	
Are my medications covered?		
How are non-covered medications approved?		
What tier/price do non-covered medications fall into once approved?		
Is Mail Order offered?		
Is there a Maximum Out of Pocket?	amount_____	
Would my drug cost reach the coverage gap?		
What would the cost be if my drugs reach the		

coverage gap?		
Would I leave the coverage gap?		
Are there preferred pharmacies?		
Is my usual pharmacy covered?		
Is customer service for the plan and/or mail order available 24 hours?		
If on plan, will medications change next year?		
Are there any special discounts that come with plan? (Ex: local pharmacy savings card)		

REVIEW
- ★ Know the dates you will be eligible to sign up or change plans.
- ★ Research each plan with your medications, checking for
  - ○ Coverage of your medications
  - ○ Pricing of your medications
- ★ ASK FOR HELP! If there is something you don't know or understand ask someone who can help. This will influence your health care for the next year, do not take it lightly!
  - ○ Ask your doctor for recommendations

- Check with friends and family who are on plans, do they like their current coverage
- Call the plan and ask questions of customer service

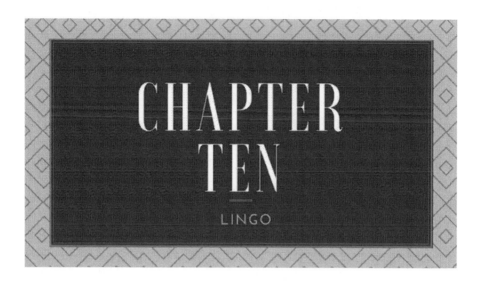

CHAPTER
TEN

LINGO

Customer: "Say what?! I don't know what you are talking about!"
Me: "Let me explain" (**Thinking, How can I make this simple)

Affordable Care Act (ACA) - Legislation passed in 2010 to lower the cost to Medicare Part D coverage gap by "closing the donut hole", added additional services to give low income individuals additional assistance; a.k.a. Obamacare

Alternative drug - Not a generic, or same active ingredient and formula, but a similar medication that may be used for the same medical therapy

Annual Enrollment Period (AEP) - Option to enroll in new plan each year. If no action taken, will continue with current plan, October 15 - December 7

Annual Notice of Change (ANOC) - Required annually to notify members of any changes to the plan for the upcoming benefit year -

may include premium, formulary, copay or coinsurance changes, mailed in September

Bridge Supply – A courtesy temporary supply of medication that plans may offer. If a mail order prescription has been sent but you have not yet received it, the mail order can ask a local pharmacy to fill a short-term supply out of your next order.

Catastrophic Coverage - Once out of the coverage gap, plan members only pay a small co-pay or coinsurance for their covered prescription for the rest of the year

Centers for Medicare & Medicaid Services (CMS) - Federal Department that oversees all Medicare programs

Co-insurance - Set percentage a plan member may be required to pay as their share of the cost for each prescription, after any deductible has been reached. Often based on tier level of plan structure.

Co-pay - Set rate amount a plan member may be required to pay as their share of the cost for each prescription, after any deductible has been reached. Often based on tier level of plan structure.

Coverage Gap - "Donut hole" temporary limit on what the drug plan will cover for the member's drugs, this changes each year until gap is closed 2020. Previous to ACA member paid full amount while in this gap

Coverage Determination - Any decision made by or on behalf of Part D plan to determine coverage of medications. Includes formulary exception, prior authorization, quantity limit, tiering exception, Part B vs D determination

Creditable Coverage - A prescription drug plan as good as or better than Medicare's

Deductible - Amount a beneficiary must pay each year for prescription before their Prescription Drug Plan begins to pay, may pertain to all or only some prescriptions

Expedite - Many requests and decisions made to the plan, members have the right/option to have these expedited

Explanation of Benefits (EOB) - Document that CMS requires Plans to mail their beneficiary each month they have a claim on their account. Will list drug usage (list of medications obtained during month), drug coverage level, Troop, Total Drug Spend, and upcoming formulary changes

Formulary - A list of drug products that will be covered by the plan sponsor, must be submitted to Medicare for approval, can have multiple tiers of pricing. If a prescription is not on the formulary, it may not be paid for by plan

Formulary Exception – A non-covered medication can be covered by the plan is certain criteria are met. A request for this exception can be made if the doctor states medicine is clinically necessary

Generic - Once a patent runs out on a prescription, other manufacturers can make the same prescription, often for a fraction of the price. This will have the same active ingredients but may contain different "filler" ingredients or impurities

Grievance - Formal complaint to a plan. Tells the plan of issues to be addressed, Medicare will often review these during audits. Can be filed with the plan or through Medicare itself. Must be filed within 60 days of incident

HIPAA - Health Insurance Portability and Accountability Act, 1996 legislation designed to keep individuals personal health information protected

Initial Drug Coverage - Initial phase of drug plan at beginning of the coverage year when copays are applied to medications, before the drug spend reaches Coverage Gap Threshold

Income Related Monthly Adjustment Amount (IRMAA) - Additional amount paid monthly on top of premium, based on income that exceeds $85,000 for individuals or $170,000 for jointly filing couples

Late Enrollment Period (LEP) - Fee for not being enrolled in a Medicare prescription drug plan, in addition to your monthly premium, added on for each month you are uncovered

Low Income Subsidy (LIS/LICS) - Extra Help, provided by CMS to those with limited income and resources. Amount of extra help depends on members income and asset level, will pay reduced or no premium, have reduced or eliminated out-of-pocket expenses, no coverage gap, Special Election Period monthly, apply with Medicare or Social Security.

Medigap - Extra health insurance you have the option to buy from private insurance companies to provide additional coverage of costs not covered by Medicare

Maximum Out of Pocket (MOOP) - Amount a plan may have that is the maximum paid out of pocket allowed by member before plan picks up remainder of cost

Network Pharmacy – Pharmacy that contracts with the prescription drug plan to offer medications at a discounted price

Preferred Pharmacy – Included in plan as a Network pharmacy at a greater level of savings

Premium - Monthly charge a member pays to participate in Prescription Drug Plan

Prior Authorization - A medication requires specific clinical criteria be met before a drug is covered, may include but not limited to; what other medications or therapies have been tried, diagnosis, other relevant medical conditions, how prescription will be administered

Standard Pharmacy – Included in plan as a Network pharmacy, but at less of a savings

Step Therapy - Requires one or more specific drugs prior to use of more expensive or toxic drugs, start with the most cost-effective and safest drug therapy and progress to other more costly or risky therapies

Tier Structure- Plans use tiers to show which drugs are available at what price, formularies can have multiple tiers

Total Drug Spend - What you the member and the plan pays for the prescription

Transition Fill - Courtesy fill by Prescription Drug Plan to allow you time to get appropriate coverage for a medication or find alternative covered medication, allowed at start of plan or when changes are made to formulary and coverage

Quantity Limits - May be applied to a medication based on clinical safety and to avoid overutilization. May apply to number dispensed by day supply or specific quantity allowed in a specific time frame

CHAPTER ELEVEN

FINAL THOUGHTS

When I started to write this book my goal was to help one person. What I realized was, I was already helping thousands at work. Yet, I needed to find a platform to get in front of the rest of the world. The government is never going to make this an educational program nor will they ever pay for you to take any courses, because I have realized what you already knew; they just take advantage of people that cannot sort through their hoops and hurdles. I hope this book provides you with the advantage you needed to be ahead of the game. The stories are real, the effect on medicine from federal control is real, and the fact that no one will care more about your health than you is real. So get real, get educated, and protect yourself. Save money and, if you want to go above and beyond, share this knowledge to save lives.

My last words of advice - stay healthy, stay positive, stay educated, and always question.

FACT: During the time you have read this book, many people

have reached the coverage gap and have no way out. Now some cannot afford their medicines to stay alive, and know that this could have happened to you. These are the same people that thought it could never happen to them.

FINAL REVIEW

- ★ Know the costs of your medications
- ★ Understand the phases of a prescription drug plan and your costs will be
- ★ Understand your prescriptions drug plan and benefits
- ★ Know your rights

CHAPTER
TWELVE

REFERENCES & RESOURCES

> Customer: "I don't know what to do, where can I find help and information?"
> Me: "Let's find your state and see."

Medicare
1-800-MEDICARE (633-4227)
www.Medicare.gov

Social Security Administration
1-800-772-1213
www.socialsecurity.gov/prescriptionhelp

Medicaid
1-877-267-2323
www.Medicaid.gov
Contact your state: https://www.medicaid.gov/about-us/contact-us/contact-state-page.html

Senior Health Insurance Assistance Program (SHIP) offers free counseling services for Medicare members. They can assist in explaining coverage, selecting a plan, and finding additional assistance services.

Find your state's resources here:
http://www.seniorsresourceguide.com/directories/National/SHIP/

Program of All-Inclusive Care for the Elderly (PACE) is a Medicare and Medicaid program that assists with medical and in home care costs. Get information and search by state at:
https://www.medicare.gov/your-medicare-costs/help-paying-costs/pace/pace.html

State Pharmaceutical Assistance Programs are independent in each state and may help with costs of medications, specifically while you are in the coverage gap.
https://www.medicare.gov/pharmaceutical-assistance-program/state-programs.aspx

Check locally with
- Friends and family
- Community centers
- Senior Centers
- Library
- AARP
- ...and more! Watch for groups online or through the newspaper that hold free information sessions.

Insurance sales broker - I put this last because I do feel it has caveats. Use word of mouth from someone you trust, find a broker that is well informed and helpful. They should not be trying to make a sale but instead give you knowledge. Brokers can be very well informed because they know about so many plans, but this may also mean they are not as well versed in the specific details of each. Just have in the back of your mind that if a broker helps enroll you in a plan they may be earning a commission. If the information they are providing you is biased in that manner, find someone else to help you.

Made in United States
Orlando, FL
02 March 2023

30605872R00048